Table of Contents

Lesson 1 Journal..
The Truth About Teens & Drugs...............................
Lesson 2 Journal..
Alcohol: What Do You Know?................................. 7
How Alcohol Could Negatively Affect My Life 9
Lesson 3 Journal.. 10
Reasons to Be Tobacco Free 11
Lesson 4 Journal.. 12
Marijuana: Know the Facts 13
What's Your Advice About Marijuana? 15
Lesson 5 Journal.. 17
Looking at Labels.. 19
In the News 21
Lesson 6 Journal.. 23
Experimenting with Drugs: Reasons & Risks 25
Lesson 7 Journal.. 28
Opioids: Know the Facts 29
In the News Again 31
Lesson 8 Journal.. 32
What Are the Negative Consequences? 33
Drug Use & My Goal 35
Lesson 9 Journal.. 36
Influences on My Choices About Drugs 37
Lesson 10 Journal.. 38
A Letter to Myself 40
Lesson 11 Journal.. 41
Reasons to Stay Drug Free 43
Lesson 12 Journal.. 44
School Drug Policies Scavenger Hunt 45
Lesson 13 Journal.. 46
Cigarette & Vape Advertising: Then & Now 47
Sharing What You Know About Vape Advertising & Youth 49
Lesson 14 Journal.. 50
Our Counter-Advertisement 51
Lesson 15 Journal.. 52
Lesson 16 Journal.. 54
Roleplay Feedback Form 55
Lesson 17 Journal.. 56
My Drug-Free Pledge 57
Health Terms Glossary 59

© 2020 ETR. All rights reserved. Published by ETR, Scotts Valley, CA. etr.org.
This *Student Workbook* is a part of ETR's *HealthSmart* K–12 program. Title No. HS065. ISBN 978-1-56240-308-9.

Lesson 1

Student Journal
Teens & Drugs: What's the Truth?

Healthy behavior

Avoiding vaping, other tobacco products, alcohol and other drugs.

Health terms

estimate
media
norms
perceived norms
percentage

Journal entry

How do you think vaping, other tobacco products, alcohol and other drugs could be a real problem or concern for teens?

Early death can happen.
• Stomach aches, lung diseases, etc.

If your friends do something...

Does that make you more or less likely to do it too? Why?

No, I wouldn't do it, but if it's their choice to do it then I won't mind. Vaping, doing drugs, etc, is very bad for the living body.

> **Norms** – The beliefs and actual behaviors shared by and accepted within a group.
>
> **Perceived norms** – What people *think* others are doing or believe.

(continued)

Lesson 1

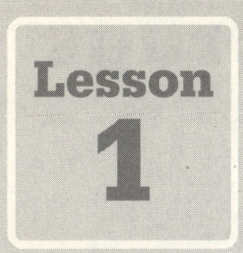

Student Journal
Teens & Drugs: What's the Truth? (continued)

Overestimating drug use

Why do you think many students overestimate the percentage of eighth graders who vape or use other tobacco products, alcohol or other drugs?

I don't know, but I'll guess because of the big problem with kids using vapes or drugs.

If a person thinks more people their age are using a drug than actually are, how might this affect their choices around drug use?

Some people might start getting influenced by this and use drugs too, but some may also do things that could help, like persuading them to stop.

My additional notes

The Truth About Teens & Drugs

Directions: Think about what you learned about teens and drugs today, and answer the questions. Be specific and give details in your answers.

▶ Part 1

Based on the data from the national survey, did most of your class guess high, guess low or accurately estimate the percent of eighth graders who are currently using each of these drugs? (Check one for each drug.)

Tobacco (cigarettes)
☑ high ☐ low ☐ accurate

Tobacco (smokeless)
☐ high ☑ low ☐ accurate

Alcohol
☐ high ☑ low ☐ accurate

Marijuana
☐ high ☑ low ☐ accurate

Vaping
☑ high ☐ low ☐ accurate

Opioids
☑ high ☐ low ☐ accurate

▶ Part 2

Many students think more young people use drugs than actually do. Why do you think this might be? Depression, Anxiety, Sleep, all those things are "reasons to take medications."

What are perceived norms? What people think other people are doing.

How can perceived norms influence a person's choices to use or not use drugs? The more people do it, the bigger the influence. Some teenagers take it because others take it, but some just persuade others to stop. Influencing someone can go two ways, the good way, or the bad way.

(continued)

The Truth About Teens & Drugs
(continued)

▶ Part 3

You have your own blog. You want people to know the truth about teens and drugs. Write a paragraph to post on your blog that explains that most teens do not vape, smoke cigarettes, use smokeless tobacco, drink alcohol or use other drugs. Use the national survey data you learned about in class to support your post.

Ya'll, we need to stop doing drugs. I just found out that teenagers don't actually do so much drugs. There is a low percentage for teens to take drugs. Perceived norms are things that people think other people are doing. Because of these "perceived norms", many teenagers think that other many teenagers are doing drugs. This makes more teenagers do drugs. Back to how there aren't actually many teenagers who do drugs, the national survey data shows also that, not many teens are not taking drugs.

This is why, we need to stop doing drugs.

Self-Check
- ☐ I reported whether the class estimates were high, low or accurate and explained why this might be.
- ☐ I defined perceived norms.
- ☐ I explained how perceived norms can influence a person's choices about drug use.
- ☐ I explained that most teens do not use drugs, using the national survey data for support.

Lesson 2

Student Journal
Alcohol: What's the Truth?

Healthy behavior

Not experimenting with or using alcohol.

Health terms

addiction
alcohol
consequences
dangers
depressant
experimentation
long term
risk
short term
stimulant

Journal entry

Write 1 thing you think you know about alcohol.

You get drunk if you drink too much.

Write 1 question you have about alcohol.

What's it made out of?

My additional notes

Alcohol: What Do You Know?

Directions: Read each statement. Put a T next to the statement if you think it is true. Put an F next to the statement if you think it is false. On the lines below each statement, explain why you think it's true or false.

T or F?

__T__ **1** Alcohol can change how the brain works.
Getting Drunk ↗↗

__F__ **2** Drinking alcohol isn't connected to doing other dangerous or risky behaviors.
Drunk driving is a good example, after having alcohol it's hard to drive since your mind is everywhere so you can get into car crashes.

__T__ **3** Alcohol is a stimulant or "upper."

__T__ **4** Alcohol can kill you.
Car crashes or too much alcohol can affect your health and make you a risk in death.

__T__ **5** Drinking alcohol can make you gain weight.
Yes. It's "scientifically" proven.

(continued)

Tobacco, Alcohol & Other Drug Prevention • Student Workbook • Lesson 2

Alcohol: What Do You Know?
(continued)

__T__ **6)** People who begin to drink alcohol before age 15 are more likely to get addicted than those who begin at the legal age of 21 or later.

It means your used to alcohol

__T__ **7)** Most teens don't drink alcohol.

Who would?

__T__ **8)** Teens who drink a lot have the same long-term health risks as adults who drink a lot.

__F__ **9)** Experimenting with alcohol can be dangerous.

Depends on how to experiment with alcohol, since alcohol isn't very dangerous like poison ivy.

__T__ **10)** Activities teens like to do can be negatively affected by drinking alcohol.

How Alcohol Could Negatively Affect My Life

Directions: Think about what you learned today about alcohol. In Part 1 write 3 negative consequences of alcohol use for teens. Next to each consequence you list, write how that consequence could negatively affect your own life, including your goals and the things you like to do. Then answer the question in Part 2. Be specific in all your answers.

▶ Part 1

Negative Consequences

1. Addiction
2. can get hurt.
3. Depression.

How It Would Affect My Life

1. People won't like me.
2. Getting drunk means losing your mind, and a higher chance to get hurt.
3. Alcohol can also effect behavior. most alcohol drinkers get in to stress or depression.

▶ Part 2

How can alcohol increase the dangerous risks a person takes? Give at least 2 specific examples of risks someone who's under the influence of alcohol might take.

Drunk driving can get you into dangerous car crashes or unsteady driving. Being drunk means losing your mind, so alcohol can get you to do bad things.

Self-Check
- ☐ I identified 3 negative consequences of alcohol use.
- ☐ I wrote a specific way each consequence could affect my life, including my goals or the things I like to do.
- ☐ I explained how alcohol can increase the risks a person takes and gave 2 specific examples.

Lesson 3

Student Journal
Vaping & Other Tobacco Products: What's the Truth?

Healthy behavior

Avoiding using or experimenting with vaping or any other tobacco product.

Health terms

addictive
bronchitis
e-cigarette
emphysema
experimentation
long term
nicotine
secondhand smoke
short term
smokeless tobacco ←
tobacco
vape device
vaping

Journal entry

Name as many different tobacco products as you can think of.

~~I know but I forgot their names~~
• Cigars • Cigarettes • Vapes • Weed gummys

How could it affect me?

Write 1 way you think vaping or using other tobacco products could negatively affect your goals or the things you like to do.

Vaping increases your anxiety and depression easily. It can make you not want to do things at all.

My additional notes

What is this???

Reasons to Be Tobacco Free

Directions: Write about what you've learned today about the negative effects of using all forms of tobacco, including vaping, and what the benefits of being tobacco free would be for you. Be clear and specific in all of your answers. In your work:
- Identify at least 3 short-term and 2 long-term negative health effects of using tobacco.
- Discuss at least 1 negative health effect of secondhand smoke.
- Discuss at least 2 negative effects of vaping.
- Describe at least 2 benefits that being tobacco and vape free would have for you.

▶ **Negative effects of using tobacco:**

Short term: _____

Long term: _____

▶ **Negative effects of secondhand smoke:**

▶ **Negative effects of vaping:**

▶ **Benefits of being tobacco free:**

Self-Check
- ☐ I identified at least 3 specific negative short-term and 2 negative long-term consequences of using tobacco.
- ☐ I discussed at least 1 specific health effect of secondhand smoke.
- ☐ I discussed at least 2 negative effects of vaping.
- ☐ I described at least 2 benefits of being tobacco free for me.

Lesson 4

Student Journal
Marijuana: What's the Truth?

Healthy behavior

Avoiding using or experimenting with marijuana.

Health terms

addiction
dependence
hallucinogen
immune system
impaired
long term
marijuana
motivation
nausea
reproductive system
short term

Journal entry

Write down 1 of the personal benefits of being drug free. Describe how it would feel to enjoy this benefit and how it would help you in your life.

I'm not mentally ill and people like me without drugs :)

Marijuana and my life

How could using marijuana negatively affect your life today in the short term, or affect your life in the future?

I get high, and when people see that, they'll call me jobless, useless, homeless, wasted, garbage, stinky poop, etc.

What do you think is the most important reason to avoid using marijuana?

It gives you illusional depression and it's not good for you.

12 Tobacco, Alcohol & Other Drug Prevention • Student Workbook • Lesson 4

Marijuana: Know the Facts

▶ What is marijuana?

Marijuana comes from the dried flowers and leaves of the cannabis plant. It's also called weed, pot, grass, dope or cannabis. It can be smoked by rolling it a cigarette, adding it to a cigar or using a pipe. It can also be mixed in foods or brewed as a tea. Marijuana or a concentrate made from the oils in the plant can also be vaped.

The drug in marijuana is called THC. THC is a mind-altering compound that changes how the brain works. It attaches to receptors in the brain that send messages to nerve cells in the body that can affect learning, memory, appetite, coordination and feelings of pleasure. The effects can vary based on how much a person uses and how long the drug is used. THC is considered a mild hallucinogen because it can alter a person's awareness and senses.

The amount of THC in marijuana determines how strong it is and how much it affects the body. Much of the marijuana grown today has a greater THC content than it did in the past. THC can stay in the body as long as a month after one use.

THC can be extra tricky when people eat marijuana. Edible marijuana products are often stronger than the marijuana people smoke, but it can take longer to feel the effects. This makes it harder to know how much THC they've eaten, and easy to eat too much.

▶ If marijuana is legal, does that mean it's safe?

Under federal law, it is still illegal to use, possess or grow marijuana. Some states have made it legal to use marijuana for treatment of certain medical conditions, and some allow adults age 21 and over to buy marijuana for personal, private use. Marijuana is illegal everywhere for people under age 21.

But just because marijuana is legal in some places, doesn't mean it's safe. Tobacco and alcohol are both legal for adult use, and the negative health effects of these two drugs are well known. Marijuana can be used to relieve some medical symptoms, such as easing nausea and vomiting in cancer patients. But marijuana can also cause negative health effects.

Short-Term Effects

These things can happen while using or shortly after, even the first time someone tries marijuana:

■ Problems with learning or short-term memory	■ Slower reflexes, being clumsy	■ Feeling worried or paranoid
■ Changes in how things look, sound or feel	■ Faster heart rate	■ Sleep problems
■ Finding it harder to pay attention	■ Dry mouth and throat, red eyes if smoking	■ Poisoning from too much THC

(continued)

Marijuana: Know the Facts
(continued)

Long-Term Effects

These things can happen over time, if a person keeps using marijuana:

- **Damage to the lungs.** Marijuana smoke can harm lung tissue and cause scaring. A person who smokes marijuana regularly can have many of the same breathing problems as people who smoke cigarettes, such as a cough and greater risk of infections. Marijuana smoke contains many of the same toxins and things that cause cancer as tobacco smoke. Vaping marijuana or THC can also cause serious damage to the lungs.

- **Heart problems.** Use of marijuana can increase or even double the heart rate. Secondhand marijuana smoke can affect the heart and blood vessels as much as secondhand tobacco smoke.

- **Brain development.** When teens begin using marijuana, it can have permanent effects because their brains are still developing. Use of the drug may reduce attention, memory, learning and problem-solving skills. It can also affect the way the brain builds connections between the parts that control these functions.

- **Mental health problems.** Frequent use or use in high doses can cause feelings of anxiety, paranoia or temporary psychosis (not knowing what is real). Marijuana use has also been linked to depression in teens. Research has found that people who use marijuana regularly for a long time are less happy with their lives.

- **Addiction.** Some marijuana users do become dependent or even addicted. For people who start using the drug before age 18 the risk is greater. Withdrawal symptoms can include feeling irritable, trouble sleeping, anxiety and craving the drug. A person might be addicted if they can't quit using, give up activities with friends and family so they can use, and continue to use marijuana even when it cause problems at home, school or work.

▶ What about young people and marijuana?

One of the biggest risks for teens is how marijuana can affect the developing brain. Because marijuana can dull attention, memory and learning, it can affect how well a person does in school. Students who use marijuana may get lower grades and be more likely to drop out of school. The effects on coordination and timing can affect how well a person does at sports.

Most teens don't use marijuana. In fact, more than 93% of eighth graders and 80% of all high school students do not use it.

Sources: Centers for Disease Control and Prevention. 2018. Marijuana and Public Health. www.cdc.gov/marijuana/index.htm; National Institute on Drug Abuse. 2017. Marijuana: Facts for Teens. www.drugabuse.gov/publications/marijuana-facts-teens/some-things-to-think-about; NIDA for Teens. 2019. Marijuana. https://teens.drugabuse.gov/drug-facts/marijuana.

What's Your Advice About Marijuana?

Directions: These are questions some fifth graders really asked. Read each letter and use what you learned about marijuana from the **Marijuana: Know the Facts** reading sheet to answer the question.
- In each of your responses to letters 1, 2 and 3, be sure to describe at least 1 negative short-term and 1 negative long-term effect of using marijuana related to the letter writer's situation.
- In your response to letter 4, clearly state in a convincing way that most teen do not use marijuana using evidence you learned from the reading.

Dear Expert,

I heard that marijuana was a safe drug to use and won't hurt your health. Is that true?

Signed,
  Confused

① Dear Confused,
Your name says a lot of things. (No offense) Though marijuana is legal in some places, it isn't healthy. It can cause damage to lungs, heart problems, slow brain development, etc. Your death ~~will fall~~ percentage will go higher.
  Signed,
  Mika

Dear Expert,

My older sister smokes pot. She's always trying to get me to try it. She tells me there's nothing wrong with it, and you can stop using anytime you want. What should I say to her?

Signed,
  Looking for Answers

② Dear Looking for Answers,
Tell her, "stop, don't talk to me, loser, lamo, wannabe, like oh, totally, totally." Smoking pot is BAD, and you will never get boyfriend / girlfriend with that bad breath if you smoke pot.
  Signed,
  Mika

(continued)

Tobacco, Alcohol & Other Drug Prevention • Student Workbook • Lesson 4   15

What's Your Advice About Marijuana?
(continued)

Dear Expert,

Two guys at the skateboard park are always talking about getting high. If I started using marijuana, would it relax me and make me a better skateboarder?

Signed,
　Inquisitive Skateboarder

3 Dear Inquisitive Skateboarder,

No. In fact, you would break your skateboard. Getting high means to go crazy, not to relax.

　　　　Signed,
　　　　Mika

Dear Expert,

I hear that almost everyone in eighth grade smokes pot. Is that true?

Signed,
　Wanting to Know the Truth

4 Dear Wanting to Know the Truth,

Understand that those are just rumors, and do not consider smoking anything but the steam from dumplings.

　　　　Signed,
　　　　Mika

Self-Check
- [ ] I described at least 1 negative short-term and 1 negative long-term effect of using marijuana in my responses to letters 1, 2 and 3.
- [ ] I described different effects in each response.
- [ ] I clearly stated that most teens do not use marijuana in my response to letter 4, using what I learned.

Lesson 5

Student Journal
Medicines: What's the Truth?

Healthy behavior

Avoiding misuse and abuse of over-the-counter and prescription drugs.

Health terms

antibiotic

antihistamine

asthma

infection

misuse

over-the-counter drug

pharmacist

prescription

Journal entry

Can you think of some drugs that can help people stay healthy or feel better when they are sick or injured?

Tylenol, Anasthesia, or just bandages or casts. Those are the safe drugs to healing.

> **Medicines** – Drugs that are used to help the body heal, relieve pain or keep certain diseases under control.
>
> **Over-the-counter drugs** – Medicines you can buy at a store without permission from a doctor.
>
> **Prescription drugs** – Medicines that you need written permission from a doctor or other licensed health care provide to take, and that must be given out by a pharmacist.

Medicine misuse

Can you think of some ways over-the-counter and prescription medicines could be misused?

Sleep meds, people who can't sleep usually take these but sometimes go crazy if they use the one that isn't right for them.

(continued)

Tobacco, Alcohol & Other Drug Prevention • Student Workbook • Lesson 5

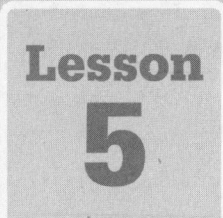

Student Journal
Medicines: What's the Truth? (continued)

Rules for taking medicines

1. Always, read the label.

2.

3.

My additional notes

Looking at Labels

Directions: Look at these sample labels for an over-the-counter medicine and a prescription medicine. Then answer the questions about each medicine.

▶ Over-the-Counter Medicine

This is a medicine used for allergies. (Antihistamines help stop itching and sneezing.)

Drug Facts

Active Ingredient (in each tablet) — **Purpose**
Chlorpheniramine maleate 2 mg...................Antihistimine

Uses temporarily relieves these symptoms due to hay fever or other upper respiratory allergies:
- sneezing ■ runny nose ■ itchy, watery eyes ■ itchy throat

Warnings
Ask a doctor before use if you have
- glaucoma ■ a breathing problem such as emphysema or chronic bronchitis
- trouble urinating due to an enlarged prostate gland

Ask a doctor or pharmacist before use if you are taking tranquilizers or sedatives

When using this product
- you may get drowsy
- alcohol, sedatives, and tranquilizers may increase drowsiness
- be careful when driving a motor vehicle or operating machinery
- excitability may occur, especially in children

If pregnant or breast-feeding, ask a health professional before use.
Keep out of reach of children. In case of overdose, get medical help or contact a Poison Control Center right away.

Directions

adults and children 12 years and over	take 2 tablets every 4 to 6 hours; not more than 12 tablets in 24 hours
children 6 years to under 12 years	take 1 tablet every 4 to 6 hours; not more than 6 tablets in 24 hours
children under 6 years	ask a doctor

Other information store at 20–25° C (68–77° F) ■ protect from excessive moisture

Inactive ingredients D&C yellow no. 10, lactose, magnesium stearate, microcrystalline cellulose, pregelatanized starch

① Under what circumstances should a person take this over-the-counter medicine?
If they have hay fever or other upper respiratory allergies

② At what time(s) should the person take this medicine?
If they have sneezing, runny nose, itchyness, watery eyes, or itchy throats.

③ What is the right amount of this medicine to take?
Two tablets / one tablet every 4-6 hours

④ How much medicine can the person take in a day?
Not more than 6/12

⑤ What are some possible side effects from taking this medicine?
Drowsiness

(continued)

Looking at Labels
(continued)

▶ Prescription Medicine

This is an antibiotic that's used to cure or prevent infection.

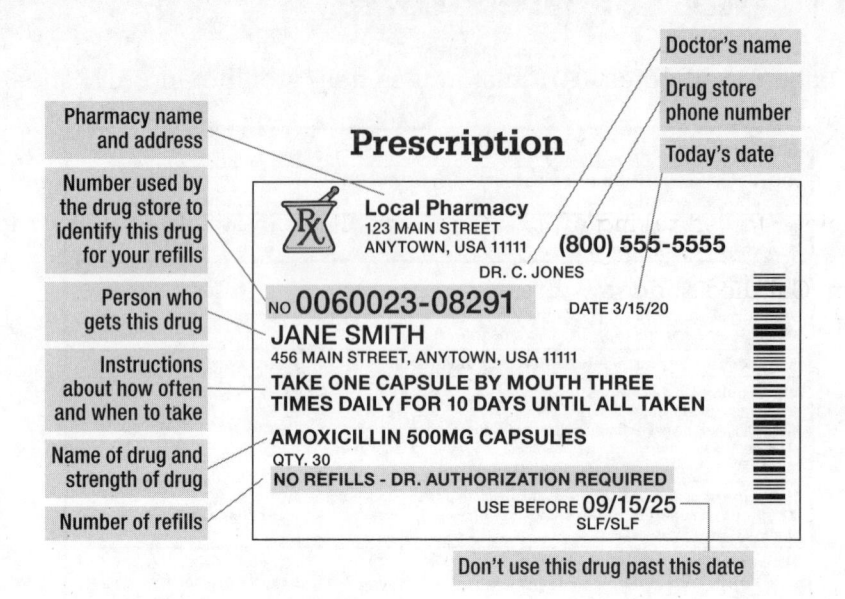

Label callouts:
- Pharmacy name and address
- Number used by the drug store to identify this drug for your refills
- Person who gets this drug
- Instructions about how often and when to take
- Name of drug and strength of drug
- Number of refills
- Doctor's name
- Drug store phone number
- Today's date
- Don't use this drug past this date

Prescription

Local Pharmacy
123 MAIN STREET
ANYTOWN, USA 11111
(800) 555-5555
DR. C. JONES
NO 0060023-08291 DATE 3/15/20
JANE SMITH
456 MAIN STREET, ANYTOWN, USA 11111
TAKE ONE CAPSULE BY MOUTH THREE TIMES DAILY FOR 10 DAYS UNTIL ALL TAKEN
AMOXICILLIN 500MG CAPSULES
QTY. 30
NO REFILLS - DR. AUTHORIZATION REQUIRED
USE BEFORE 09/15/25
SLF/SLF

① Who would be the right person to take this prescription medicine?
Jane Smith

② At what time(s) should the person take this medicine?
Three times daily for 10 days

③ What is the right amount of this medicine to take?
One capsule

④ How much medicine can the person take in a day?
Three

⑤ How long should the person take this medicine?
For 10 days (ten)

Self-Check
☐ I answered all of the questions for the over-the-counter medicine.
☐ I answered all of the questions for the prescription medicine.

In the News

Directions: The information in these stories is true. The names of the teens have been changed to protect their identities. Read each story and decide whether it is an example of proper use or misuse and explain why based on the details in the story. Then describe the negative effects of each type of drug.

▶ Cal

Cal, a 17-year-old senior, started taking a friend's prescription painkillers to help deal with some back pain. Cal died suddenly after mixing over-the-counter cold medicine and the friend's painkillers. Cal's father said that Cal wasn't aware of the dangers of prescription drugs because they were legal drugs.

Is this an example of proper use or misuse?
misuse

Why? Cal died, and the painkiller wasn't for him.

▶ Justin

Justin was a nationally ranked high school tennis player. His parents had no idea their son was going to school and to practice high on prescription drugs. Justin started stealing and using prescription drugs when he was just 13 years old. By the time Justin was 17, he was losing a lot of weight and looking sick, and his parents finally checked him into a drug treatment clinic. Because of his drug addiction, Justin missed most of his senior year in high school and lost his national ranking as a tennis player.

Is this an example of proper use or misuse?
misuse

Why? He was stealing prescription bottles that weren't right for him and got even sicker.

▶ Sharise

Sharise assumed that all over-the-counter medicines were safe. She took aspirin for a headache and cough syrup when she had a cold and never had any problems. So when her best friend told her she could take a lot of cough syrup to get high, Sharise thought it wouldn't be a big deal. But after she drank a large amount of cough syrup all at once, she began to feel dizzy and nauseous, and started having a seizure. Sharise's friend got scared and told her mom. They took Sharise to the emergency room.

Is this an example of proper use or misuse?
misuse

Why? Though cough syrup is okay, it's not good to take so much at once.

(continued)

In the News (continued)

▶ Kaitlyn

Kaitlyn, a middle school student, hurt her back during gymnastics practice. Her coach told her to ice her back and skip practice for a few days. Kaitlyn did this, but her back still hurt, so her mom took her to their family doctor for help. The doctor prescribed a pain medicine. Kaitlyn and her mom picked up the prescription from the pharmacy and read the directions together. Kaitlyn followed the directions on the label and took the medicine twice a day for a few days. After a week, her back started to feel better and Kaitlyn was able to go to gymnastics again.

Is this an example of proper use or misuse? _proper_

Why? _Kaitlyn read the label, used the medicine that was prescribed for her, and followed the directions._

▶ Angel

Angel had a cold a few weeks ago. The other symptoms cleared up, but Angel was still coughing 3 weeks later. When the cough kept getting worse, not better, Angel went to the doctor. The doctor said that Angel had developed an infection and prescribed antibiotics to take 3 times a day. After a few days, the cough was nearly gone and Angel was feeling much better. Angel thought about not taking the rest of the medicine. But the directions that came with the prescription said to keep taking the prescribed dose until the pills were all gone. So Angel kept taking the antibiotic for the full 10 days.

Is this an example of proper use or misuse? _proper_

Why? _Angel followed the directions of the prescription and will heal better as ever._

Describe the negative effects (physical, emotional, social) of misusing:

Prescription medicines _get high, get sick, get weak, may die if using any other medicine._

Over-the-counter medicines _if you take too much, you can get very nauseous, and if you take while you're not sick, you're in trouble (in a medical way)_

Self-Check
☐ I determined whether each story showed proper use or misuse of the drug and explained why.
☐ I described the negative effects of misusing each type of medicine.

Lesson 6

Student Journal
Experimentation & Addiction: What's the Truth?

Healthy behavior

Avoiding experimenting with vaping, other tobacco products, alcohol and other drugs.

Health terms

addiction
denial
dependence
experimentation
stages
tolerance
withdrawal

Journal entry

What does it mean to *experiment* with something?

Try (something)

Is experimenting always a good thing? Can it ever be bad? Or does it depend? Explain why.

No, not always, experiments could always contain something dangerous, like, lets say you're experimenting drugs on yourself. Dangerous? I think so too.

Why is it dangerous to experiment with any kind of drug?

It could give you cancer, diseases, heart problems, or anything that can shorten your life.

(continued)

Tobacco, Alcohol & Other Drug Prevention • Student Workbook • Lesson 6   23

Lesson 6

Student Journal
Experimentation & Addiction: What's the Truth? *(continued)*

Stages of addiction

1. _____

2. _____

3. _____

4. _____

5. _____

My additional notes

Experimenting with Drugs: Reasons & Risks

Directions: Each of these case studies shows someone in a different stage of addiction. For each one, answer the questions about why the person started using the drug and what risks or consequences are happening because of the drug use.

Stages of Addiction

1. **First use** The person tries a drug for the first time.
2. **Continued use** The person keeps using the drug to feel a certain way.
3. **Tolerance** It takes more of the drug to get high.
4. **Dependence** The person gets sick without the drug.
5. **Addiction** The person can't stop using the drug, even when the drug use causes serious problems.

▶ Case Study 1

"I started using chewing tobacco a few years ago when my older brother gave me some. It was fun to hang out with him and his friends and I liked how it made me feel. But lately everybody's getting on my case! I asked my best friend if I could borrow some money for chew and he told me he's going to stop hanging out with me if I keep using it. Who cares? I don't need him as a friend! And my mom's mad at me because she found a tin in the back pocket of the jeans I put in the wash. She's bugging me to quit too. This morning I saw a weird white spot in my mouth. But I know that if I tell anyone, they're going to hassle me about using tobacco. So I'm just going to wait and see if it gets better. It's probably nothing to worry about."

Why did this person start using smokeless tobacco? *I'm guessing because he thought chewing tobacco was better than smoking.*

What risks or consequences are happening because of the drug use? *You can get high and your breath could STANK.*

▶ Case Study 2

"I've been having a beer a few times a week. My dad always has it around, so it's easy to take one without him noticing. I first tried it before midterms and it helped me feel more relaxed and less worried about school and stuff. But I don't drink that much—just when I'm feeling stressed and need to relax and calm down. I know it's becoming more of a habit, but I'll stop or cut back once life isn't so stressful anymore."

Why did this person start drinking alcohol? *Because this guy has stress.*

Why is using alcohol or other drugs an unhealthy way to manage stress? *Because it can make you more stressful.*

(continued)

Experimenting with Drugs: Reasons & Risks *(continued)*

▶ Case Study 3

"I first tried vaping because I saw some posts on social media that made it look cool. I kept doing it because I liked it. I guess I've been doing it more often lately, but I didn't think it would be a big deal to stop for a while. We went to my grandma's house for the weekend and she's really strict. Since my granddad died of lung cancer a few years ago, she won't let anyone smoke or vape at her house—not even outside. So I left my JUUL at home because I didn't want her to get mad if she found it. That was a mistake. I got this bad headache and felt really cranky the whole weekend. It was hard to sleep at night too."

Why did this person start vaping? _____

_____

What risks or consequences are happening because of the drug use? _____

_____

▶ Case Study 4

"I like to drink beer at parties. It helps me have fun, feel less shy and act more social. So I've been having a few beers whenever I go to a party on the weekend. But lately I'm just not getting the same kind of buzz from it. This weekend I'm hoping there's some stronger kind of alcohol at the party. I'm going to switch to tequila or some other liquor and see if that gives me those same feelings again."

Why did this person start drinking alcohol? _____

_____

What risks or consequences are happening because of the drug use? _____

_____

(continued)

Experimenting with Drugs: Reasons & Risks *(continued)*

▶ Case Study 5

"These guys I skateboard with started using marijuana. I know it's not supposed to be good for you, but it's not like it's illegal anymore. Plus, they're cool and I like hanging out with them. I was curious about what it was like. So one day when they offered me a joint, I took a drag. I thought I was going to cough my lungs out. But then I got this buzz that felt pretty good…"

Why did this person decide to try marijuana? _____

_____

What risks or consequences could this lead to? _____

_____
_____

Why is it dangerous to experiment with vaping, other tobacco products, alcohol or other drugs? (Support your answer with at least 1 example from the case studies.)

_____
_____
_____
_____
_____
_____
_____
_____
_____
_____

Self-Check
- ☐ I listed at least 1 reason the person in each case study started using drugs.
- ☐ I described a risk or consequence of drug use for each case study.
- ☐ I explained why experimenting with drugs is dangerous and included at least one example.

Tobacco, Alcohol & Other Drug Prevention • Student Workbook • Lesson 6

Lesson 7

Student Journal
Opioids: What's the Truth?

Healthy behavior

Avoiding misuse of the prescription drugs known as opioids.

Health terms

heroin
misuse
narcotic
opioid
overdose
tolerance

Journal entry

Drug addiction can cause many problems in a person's life.

List at least 2 of those problems or negative consequences.

_____
_____
_____
_____

> **Opioids** – Prescription drugs that are used to relieve pain.

What do you think...

is the biggest risk of opioid misuse?

_____
_____
_____
_____

My additional notes

_____
_____
_____
_____
_____
_____

Opioids: Know the Facts

Directions: Listen as the first section is read aloud. Then read the other sections on your own. As you read, take notes on what you think are the two most important pieces of information or key points in each section of the reading.

What are opioids?

Opioids are a type of drug. They include prescription medicines that are used to relieve pain.

If you've ever had a sports injury, dental work or surgery, you might have been prescribed an opioid by a doctor.

How do opioids work?

Opioids work by blocking pain receptors in the brain, which keeps a person from feeling pain. This is why they are often prescribed after surgery or for serious injuries or illness. They also trigger the release of a chemical that causes the person to feel good and happy. But these feelings don't last, which makes the brain want more of the drug.

This starts a dangerous cycle. Even if the pills were originally prescribed for pain relief, the person starts to need the drug just to feel normal.

Over time, opioids can change how the brain works. The person develops tolerance, which means they need more of the drug to get the same effects. If the person stops taking the opioid, it can be uncomfortable and painful. This makes it very hard to stop using the drug and is why opioids are so addictive.

Key points: _____

_____

_____

_____

_____

_____

Sources: NIDA for Teens, https://teens.drugabuse.gov/drug-facts/prescription-pain-medications-opioids; Truth Initiative, https://opioids.thetruth.com.

(continued)

Opioids: Know the Facts
(continued)

What is opioid misuse?

Most people begin using opioids when they get a prescription from a doctor to control pain. When opioids are used the way they were prescribed they can be helpful for managing pain and can help people recover from surgery or injuries.

But it's easy to misuse opioids. A person misuses these drugs when they:

- Take more of the medicine than was prescribed.
- Take the medicine more often than what was prescribed.
- Take the medicine longer than they're supposed to.
- Take opioids that weren't prescribed for them.
- Take opioids to get high.

Key points: _____
_____
_____
_____
_____

What are the negative consequences of opioid misuse?

When people who have become addicted to opioids can no longer get a prescription for them, they often begin using illegal drugs, such as heroin, to get the same effects.

Opioid misuse can lead to all the negative consequences that come with addiction. The person can't stop using opioids, even when the drug use causes serious problems with their health or other aspects of their life.

Overdose is a very big risk with opioid use. Because opioids affect the part of the brain that controls breathing, taking too much of an opioid can lead to emergency room visits and even death.

Key points: _____
_____
_____
_____
_____

In the News Again

Directions: Read the story and answer the questions.

Kaitlyn and Bryce

Kaitlyn, a middle school student, hurt her back during gymnastics practice. Her coach told her to ice her back and skip practice for a few days. Kaitlyn did this, but her back still hurt, so her mom took her to the clinic for help.

The doctor at the clinic prescribed an opioid pain medicine. Kaitlyn and her mom picked up the prescription from the pharmacy and read the directions together. Kaitlyn followed the directions on the label and took the medicine twice a day for a few days. After a week, her back started to feel much better and Kaitlyn was able to go to gymnastics again.

Kaitlyn's friend Bryce is also on the gymnastics team. Right before an important meet, Bryce twisted an ankle during a routine. Bryce said it really hurt and was upset about missing the meet because of the injury. Kaitlyn still had some of the medicine the doctor had prescribed for her back, so she gave one of the leftover pills to Bryce.

Bryce took the pill and was able to compete in the meet. "That pill was great," Bryce told Kaitlyn later. "It took the pain away and made me feel really good!"

The next day, Bryce asked if Kaitlyn had any more of the pills. Kaitlyn wasn't sure it was a good idea to share them, but Bryce said it was "just in case I hurt myself before a meet again." Kaitlyn's back injury was healed and she felt fine, plus she wanted to make her friend happy, so she gave the rest of the pills to Bryce.

What is an example of proper use from the story? _____

_____

What is an example of misuse from the story? _____

_____

What could happen if Bryce keeps using the pain pills from Kaitlyn? Write an ending to the story that describes at least 1 negative consequence of misusing opioids.

_____
_____
_____
_____
_____
_____

Self-Check
☐ I identified examples of proper use and misuse.
☐ I wrote an ending that describes at least 1 negative consequence.

Lesson 8

Student Journal
Consequences of Drug Use: How Bad Could It Be?

Healthy behavior

Avoiding using or experimenting with vaping, other tobacco products, alcohol and other drugs.

Health terms

consequences
facilitator
financial
legal
negative
physical
social

Journal entry

When you hear the word "consequence" what do you think of?

_____
_____
_____
_____
_____
_____

Consequences can be positive or negative

Can you think of an action, choice or behavior that resulted in a positive consequence for you?

_____
_____
_____
_____

What about one that had a negative consequence?

_____
_____
_____
_____

My additional notes

_____
_____
_____
_____
_____

What Are the Negative Consequences?

Directions: For each area, write the 3 most likely consequences of drug use that the group for that area reports. Rate how serious you think each consequence is and explain your ratings.

How serious is it?
Not ←——————→ Very

Physical/Body	0	1	2	3	4
1					
2					
3					
Explain your ratings:					

Family	0	1	2	3	4
1					
2					
3					
Explain your ratings:					

Friends	0	1	2	3	4
1					
2					
3					
Explain your ratings:					

School/Work	0	1	2	3	4
1					
2					
3					
Explain your ratings:					

(continued)

What Are the Negative Consequences?

(continued)

How serious is it?
Not ⟵⟶ Very

Legal/Law	0	1	2	3	4
1					
2					
3					

Explain your ratings:

Financial	0	1	2	3	4
1					
2					
3					

Explain your ratings:

Future	0	1	2	3	4
1					
2					
3					

Explain your ratings:

Self-Check
☐ I recorded 3 likely consequences of drug use for each area.
☐ I rated how serious each consequence would be.
☐ I explained my ratings.

Drug Use & My Goal

Directions: Write a goal you have for your future. Then list 3 negative consequences of experimenting with drugs. Explain how each consequence could affect your goal and why it would be serious for you.

My goal:

Consequence 1

How It Could Interfere:	Why it would be serious:

Consequence 2

How It Could Interfere:	Why it would be serious:

Consequence 3

How It Could Interfere:	Why it would be serious:

Self-Check
☐ I wrote how 3 consequences of drug use could interfere with my goal and why each would be serious.

Lesson 9

Student Journal
Influences on My Choices About Drugs

Healthy behavior

Avoiding using or experimenting with vaping, other tobacco products, alcohol and other drugs.

Health terms

analyze

environment

external influence

influence

internal influence

media

negative influence

positive influence

Journal entry

Write what you think the word *influence* means and give an example.

_____
_____
_____
_____
_____
_____

Describe a time you were influenced to do or not do something.

Influences on Choices About Drugs	
Positive Influences	Negative Influences

36   Tobacco, Alcohol & Other Drug Prevention • Student Workbook • Lesson 9

Influences on My Choices About Drugs

Directions: Use what you've learned about analyzing influences to answer the questions.

—

Describe how 2 negative influences might pressure you to experiment with or use tobacco, alcohol or other drugs.

_____
_____
_____
_____
_____
_____

+

Describe how 2 positive influences can help support you in being drug free.

_____
_____
_____
_____
_____
_____

↓

What is 1 strategy you could use to counter one of these negative influences and how would you use this strategy?

_____
_____
_____
_____
_____
_____
_____

↓

What's a positive influence that would help you avoid using drugs, and how could you strengthen or add this influence to your life?

_____
_____
_____
_____
_____
_____

Self-Check
☐ I identified how to counter a negative influence.
☐ I described how to strengthen a positive influence.

Tobacco, Alcohol & Other Drug Prevention • Student Workbook • Lesson 9

Lesson 10

Student Journal
Self-Talk for Being Drug Free

Healthy behavior

Avoiding using or experimenting with vaping, other tobacco products, alcohol and other drugs.

Health terms

counter
external influence
internal influence
self-talk

Journal entry

> **Internal influences** come from inside yourself.
> **External influences** come from the world around you.

List 1 *negative internal* influence and 1 *negative external* influence that might pressure you to experiment with vaping, other tobacco products, alcohol or other drugs.

– (Internal) _____

– (External) _____

List 1 *positive internal* influence and 1 *positive external* influence that could support you in staying drug free.

+ (Internal) _____

+ (External) _____

Suppose a friend was thinking about experimenting with vaping, other tobacco products or alcohol. What's something you could say to support your friend in staying drug free?

_____
_____
_____
_____
_____
_____
_____
_____
_____

(continued)

Lesson 10

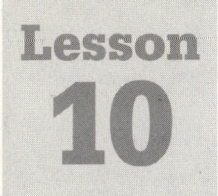

Student Journal
Self-Talk for Being Drug Free (continued)

> **Self-Talk** – The ideas that you think to yourself.

Use self-talk to counter these negative influences:
You're curious about what using marijuana feels like.
You're starting to feel as if you're the only person in your grade who hasn't been drunk.
A popular student at school just offered you a JUUL.
A friend wants you to come to a party where there will be alcohol.

A Letter to Myself

Directions: Write a letter to yourself that uses self-talk about being drug free. In your letter:
- Describe 1 negative internal influence (something from inside yourself) and explain how this might pressure you to experiment with vaping, other tobacco products, alcohol or other drugs.
- Describe at least 1 person, thing or situation that might be a negative external influence and explain how this might pressure you to experiment with vaping, other tobacco products, alcohol or other drugs.
- Write what you could say to yourself (your self-talk) to counter this negative internal influence and this negative external influence.

Dear _____,

Here's how an internal influence might pressure me to use drugs:
_____
_____

Here's how an external influence might pressure me to use drugs:
_____
_____

Here's what I can say to myself to counter these negative influences:

Internal: _____
_____
_____

External: _____
_____
_____
_____

Sincerely,

_____

Self-Check
- ☐ I explained how 1 internal influence might pressure me to use drugs.
- ☐ I explained how 1 external influence might pressure me to use drugs.
- ☐ I wrote specific self-talk I could use to counter these internal and external negative influences.

Lesson 11

Student Journal
My Peers & Their Feelings About Drugs

Healthy behavior

Avoiding using or experimenting with vaping, other tobacco products, alcohol and other drugs.

Health terms

alternative

benefit

curiosity

facilitator

peers

rebel

Journal entry

Close your eyes and imagine this situation:

> A group of popular students asked you to hang out with them after school and vape. You told them NO and walked away. Now you see the group looking over at you, whispering to each other and laughing.

Write a self-talk statement you could say to yourself that would help support your choice to stay drug free.

_____
_____
_____
_____
_____
_____

Reason Teens Might Use Drugs	Way to Address it

(continued)

Tobacco, Alcohol & Other Drug Prevention • Student Workbook • Lesson 11   41

Lesson 11

Student Journal
My Peers & Their Feelings About Drugs (continued)

Reasons Teens Would Choose Not to Use Drugs

Which of these reasons not to use drugs would be most powerful for you?

Good Things About Being Drug Free

Which of these good things would most help you stay drug free?

Reasons to Stay Drug Free

Directions: List 2 reasons teens might choose to use drugs. For each of these reasons, describe at least 2 healthy things they could do instead. Then list 3 reasons teens choose NOT to use drugs, and write your specific top 3 good things about staying drug free.

Reason Teens Might Use Drugs	Healthy Things to Do Instead
1	
2	

Reasons Teens Choose Not to Use Drugs

1
2
3

My top 3 good things about staying drug free:

1
2
3

Self-Check
☐ I listed at least 2 reasons teens might use drugs.
☐ For each reason, I wrote 2 healthy things they could do instead.
☐ I listed at least 3 reasons teens choose not to use drugs.
☐ I wrote my specific top 3 good things about staying drug free.

Lesson 12

Student Journal
Family, School & Community Rules About Drugs

Healthy behavior

Avoiding using or experimenting with vaping, other tobacco products, alcohol and other drugs, and supporting others to be drug free.

Health terms

minors

policy

possession

scavenger hunt

Journal entry

List as many drug-free alternatives as you can think of.

_____
_____
_____
_____
_____
_____
_____
_____
_____

Rules and laws

How can school rules and public laws about vaping, other tobacco products, alcohol and other drugs help keep young people drug free?

_____
_____
_____
_____
_____

My additional notes

_____
_____
_____
_____
_____

School Drug Policies Scavenger Hunt

> **Directions:** With your partner, use the student handbook to find the answers to Questions 1 through 6.

1 What are the rules about vaping or using other tobacco products on school property?

_____
_____
_____

2 What are the consequences if you are caught vaping or using other tobacco products on school property?

_____
_____
_____

3 What are the rules about using alcohol on school property?

_____
_____
_____

4 What are the consequences if you are caught using alcohol on school property?

_____
_____
_____

5 What are the rules about using other drugs on school property?

_____
_____
_____

6 What are the consequences if you are caught using other drugs on school property?

_____
_____

> **Self-Check**
> ☐ We used the school handbook to find accurate answers to all 6 questions.

Lesson 13

Student Journal
Tobacco Companies: Are They Targeting Youth?

Healthy behavior

Avoiding using or experimenting with vaping or any other tobacco product.

Health terms

advertising
industry
lawsuit
merchandise
nicotine
recruit
self-image
sponsorship
target

Journal entry

Make a list of all the negative consequences you can remember that can happen to people who vape, smoke or use smokeless tobacco.

_____
_____
_____
_____
_____
_____
_____
_____

Vape advertising and teens

Tobacco companies say they never target youth in their advertising campaigns for vaping products. Do you think this is true? Why or why not?

_____
_____
_____
_____
_____

My additional notes

_____
_____
_____
_____
_____

Cigarette & Vape Advertising: Then & Now

▶ That was then...

Before all the health risks of tobacco use were common knowledge, a lot of people smoked cigarettes. Attracting young people was important to the tobacco industry because they needed new recruits to replace the users who died or quit. The advertising techniques they used to attract teens and get them to try smoking or smokeless tobacco included sponsorship of sports events; giving away clothing, merchandise and other prizes; and creating ads that often featured cartoon characters or sweet flavors to make smoking and smokeless tobacco use look fun, exciting and social.

Lawsuits against the tobacco industry resulted in many restrictions on advertising, especially to young people. This, along with growing public awareness of the health risks and rules against smoking in public places, resulted in a decrease in tobacco use. In 1991, 27.5% of high school students had smoked during the last month. By 2017, that had dropped to only 8.8%.

Why are fewer young people smoking today?

_____
_____
_____
_____
_____
_____

▶ This is now...

Today, many young people who wouldn't dream of smoking a cigarette are curious about or willing to try vaping. What they often don't realize is that most vape juice contains nicotine, the same addictive drug as in tobacco. In fact, one JUUL pod contains as much nicotine as 1 to 2 packs of cigarettes. They also may not realize that big tobacco companies now own about 95% of the vaping market. These tobacco companies are using the same techniques that used to work for cigarette advertising to encourage a new generation to get hooked on nicotine through vaping.

The tobacco industry claimed that it didn't market its products to young people. This was disproved by company memos and letters that were disclosed during the lawsuits. Today, tobacco companies are making the same claims about their vaping marketing, saying that their products are intended to help adult smokers quit. But the flavors and ads they promote are clearly designed to appeal to young people. In fact, 43% of young people who have tried vaping say that the flavors are the main reason they started.

(continued)

Cigarette & Vape Advertising: Then & Now *(continued)*

Tobacco companies use many of the same tactics to promote vaping products that they once used for cigarettes, including offering scholarships, sponsoring music festivals and events, and introducing appealing flavors. They also have a new recruiting technique that didn't really exist back when tobacco advertising was allowed. They try to create a buzz on social media. For example, from 2015 to 2107, the number of tweets related to JUUL skyrocketed from a monthly average of 765 to a monthly average of 30,565.

Seeing messages and images on social media contributes to the mistaken idea that many more young people vape than actually do. JUUL has paid for campaigns on Twitter, Instagram and YouTube to promote images and company-sponsored ads that associate JUUL with being cool, having fun, relaxation, freedom and sex appeal.

The tobacco industry claims its vaping marketing does not target teens. What do you think? What is your evidence?

_____
_____
_____
_____
_____
_____

If the tobacco industry succeeds in getting young people to try its vaping products, what could happen?

_____
_____
_____
_____
_____
_____

Sources:

Smithsonian, www.smithsonianmag.com/history/electronic-cigarettes-millennial-appeal-ushers-next-generation-nicotine-addicts-180968747

Open Secrets, www.opensecrets.org/news/issues/e-cigarettes

Stanford University School of Medicine, http://tobacco.stanford.edu/tobacco_main/publications/JUUL_Marketing_Stanford.pdf

Truth Initiative, www.truthinitiative.org

Self-Check
- ☐ I responded to all of the questions.
- ☐ I cited evidence from the reading to support my answers.

Sharing What You Know About Vape Advertising & Youth

Directions: Write a letter to a government official (state legislator, U.S. representative, U.S. senator) that describes at least 2 ways tobacco companies target youth. Share at least 2 facts to convince this person that the tobacco industry shouldn't be allowed to target young people with vaping marketing.

Self-Check
☐ I described at least 2 ways the tobacco industry targets youth.
☐ I shared at least 2 facts to write a convincing argument.

Lesson 14

Student Journal
Counter-Advertisements

Healthy behavior

Supporting others to avoid vaping, other tobacco products and alcohol.

Health terms

advocacy

bandwagon

counter-advertisement

manipulation

testimonial

Journal entry

List some of the things the tobacco industry does to try to get teens to vape.

_____
_____
_____
_____
_____
_____
_____
_____

Advertising strategies

Bandwagon:
_____

Beauty or Sex Appeal:
_____

Emotional Appeal:
_____

Facts and Figures:
_____

Humor:
_____

Snob Appeal:
_____

Star Appeal:
_____

Testimonial:
_____

Our Counter-Advertisement

Directions: Create your own counter-advertisement to convince young people not to start using tobacco products or alcohol. You can focus on vaping, smoking, using smokeless tobacco or drinking alcohol.

Use at least 1 of the advertising strategies and make your message appeal to teens. Share the facts in your ad. Include at least 1 negative consequence of vaping, smoking, using smokeless tobacco or drinking alcohol, and 1 benefit of being drug free.

Counter-Ad created by:

_____ and _____
           name   name

1 Which drug will we create our counter ad about?
_____

2 Which advertising strategy will we use?
_____

3 What format will we use for our ad?
- ☐ poster or meme
- ☐ 30-second video
- ☐ 5 text messages
- ☐ 3 social media posts
- ☐ other: _____

4 What negative consequence of using this drug will we include in our ad?
_____
_____

5 What benefit of being drug free will we include in our ad?
_____
_____

6 How will we make our ad appeal to teens?
_____
_____
_____
_____

Self-Check
- ☐ We included accurate information about at least 1 negative consequence of using the drug.
- ☐ We included at least 1 benefit of staying drug free.
- ☐ We used at least 1 advertising strategy in our ad.
- ☐ Our ad and its message will appeal to teens.

Lesson 15

Student Journal
Peer Pressure: Ways to Say No

Healthy behavior

Avoiding using or experimenting with vaping, other tobacco products, alcohol and other drugs.

Health terms

alternative
believable
body language
peers
pressure
resist

Journal entry

What are some situations in which a person might feel pressure to vape or use other tobacco products, alcohol or other drugs?

Pressure

How does it feel to be pressured?

Pressure lines:

(continued)

52   Tobacco, Alcohol & Other Drug Prevention • Student Workbook • Lesson 15

Lesson 15

Student Journal
Peer Pressure: Ways to Say No (continued)

Saying NO to drug pressure

Say NO:
_____
_____

Use body language and actions that support the NO message:
_____
_____

Suggest an alternative:
_____
_____

Repeat:
_____
_____

> **Make sure words and actions are real for the situation and would work with the people you know.**

My additional notes
_____
_____
_____
_____
_____
_____
_____
_____
_____

Lesson 16

Student Journal
Roleplay Practice: Resisting Drug Pressures

Healthy behavior

Avoiding using or experimenting with vaping, other tobacco products, alcohol and other drugs.

Health terms

alternative
effective
feedback
ineffective
outcome
reinforce
roleplay

Journal entry

Write about or draw a picture of a time or situation when you wanted to say NO to something, but it was hard to do. For example, were you ever pressured to go somewhere or do something with a friend that you knew you shouldn't? Describe or show how that felt.

My additional notes

Roleplay Feedback Form

Directions: As you watch the roleplays, check off the effective ways to say NO that you see in each one.

Ways to Say NO

	Roleplay 1	Roleplay 2	Roleplay 3	Roleplay 4	Roleplay 5	Roleplay 6
Said NO	☐	☐	☐	☐	☐	☐
Used a firm tone of voice	☐	☐	☐	☐	☐	☐
Body language supported the NO	☐	☐	☐	☐	☐	☐
Said NO more than once if needed	☐	☐	☐	☐	☐	☐
Suggested an alternative	☐	☐	☐	☐	☐	☐
Words and actions						
Were real for the situation	☐	☐	☐	☐	☐	☐
Would work with people you know	☐	☐	☐	☐	☐	☐

Self-Check

☐ These are the skills I did well: _____
_____
_____

☐ These are the skills I still need to work on: _____
_____
_____

Choose one and explain your answer:

☐ I feel confident I can use the skills I'm learning to say NO.

☐ I do not feel confident I can use the skills I'm learning to say NO.

_____
_____
_____

Lesson 17

Student Journal
Drug-Free Pledges: Support for Myself & Others

Healthy behavior

Avoiding using or experimenting with vaping, other tobacco products, alcohol and other drugs, and supporting others to be drug free.

Health terms

pledge

responsibility

Journal entry

Write 1 thing you can do to resist pressure to vape or use other tobacco products, alcohol or other drugs.

_____
_____
_____
_____

Pledge =

It's your choice

Why is it important to take personal responsibility for the choices you make about vaping, other tobacco products, alcohol and other drugs?

_____
_____
_____
_____

Supporting others

What are some things you can do to help everyone in the class keep their pledges?

_____
_____
_____
_____

My Drug-Free Pledge

I, _____
(Print your name.)

promise to

_____
(List something specific you will do to stay drug free.)

▶ 3 benefits or rewards of keeping my pledge:

1. _____
_____
_____

2. _____
_____
_____

3. _____
_____
_____

Signed, _____ _____
(Sign your name)   (Date)

(continued)

My Drug-Free *Pledge* (continued)

▶ **The words and actions I'll use to keep my drug-free pledge**

3 things I can say:

1. _____
_____
_____

2. _____
_____
_____

3. _____
_____
_____

3 things I can do:

1. _____
_____
_____

2. _____
_____
_____

3. _____
_____
_____

Self-Check
☐ I completed the pledge with something specific I will do to stay drug free.
☐ I described at least 3 benefits of keeping my pledge.
☐ I gave at least 3 examples of what I could say and 3 examples of what I could do to keep my pledge.

Health Terms Glossary

addiction—Physical and/or mental dependence on a drug.

addictive—Relating to or causing physical and mental dependence on a drug.

advertising—Promoting a product for sale through various media.

advertising techniques—Strategies companies use to promote their products.

advocacy—Taking planned action to have a positive effect on other people's behaviors or the environment.

alcohol—A drug formed by fermenting grains or fruits.

alternative—Something a person uses or does in place of something else.

analyze—To examine closely and use one's observations to reach a conclusion.

antibiotic—A drug used to treat infections caused by bacteria.

antihistamine—A drug used to help reduce itching and sneezing.

asthma—A disease in which the muscles around the airways tense up, the tissues that line the airways swell, and the airways produce extra mucus, making it hard to breathe and keeping the lungs from getting enough air.

bandwagon—The wagon or platform a band rides on in a parade; "getting on the bandwagon" refers to joining the popular or apparently winning side.

believable—Able to be trusted as true; possible.

benefit—Something that is advantageous or good or promotes well-being.

body language—The gestures, facial expressions and other physical clues that go with and can reinforce a verbal message; what a person is saying nonverbally with their body.

bronchitis—Inflammation of the main air passages to the lungs.

consequences—The results or outcomes of an action or event.

counter—To go against or oppose something.

counter-advertisement—An ad that discourages people from buying or using a product.

curiosity—A desire to learn or find out about something.

dangers—Things that may injure or pose a threat to a person's health or well-being.

denial—Refusing to admit to something. It's a sign of addiction when a user won't admit that drug use is causing problems in their life.

dependence—A state in which the body relies on the effect produced by a drug; may be physical or mental.

Health Terms Glossary

(continued)

depressant—A drug that slows down the central nervous system.

drug—A chemical substance, natural or human made, that alters normal body functions in some way.

effective—Producing a desired effect; working well.

emphysema—A disease caused by damage to the alveoli or air sacs in the lungs; causes shortness of breath.

environment—All the things and conditions that surround and affect a person.

estimate—To guess or calculate a number or amount.

experimentation—Trying something, such as a drug, to find out what will happen.

external influence—Things outside a person that affect their attitudes, beliefs and behaviors; can include family, peers, media and the environment.

facilitator—A person who makes things easier, such as in a group discussion.

feedback—Constructive comments about how to improve an activity or skill.

financial—Having to do with money.

hallucinogen—A drug that alters users' perceptions, making them see or hear things that aren't really there.

immune system—The body's system of defense against disease, made up of special cells and proteins in the blood and other body fluids.

impaired—Damaged or diminished in strength.

industry—A specific branch of manufacturing, or all of these collectively; any large-scale business activity.

ineffective—Failing to produce a desired effect; not working well.

infection—A disease caused by bacteria, a virus or other pathogen; sometimes passed from one person to another.

influence—Things that affect a person's attitudes, beliefs or behaviors; can be positive or negative.

internal influence—Things from inside a person that affect their attitudes, beliefs and behaviors; can include feelings, personal experiences and self-talk.

Health Terms Glossary

(continued)

lawsuit—A case in a court of law involving a claim or complaint by one party against another.

legal—Having to do with the law.

long term—Happening over time.

manipulation—The act of tricking or convincing someone to believe or act in certain ways, often by unfair means.

marijuana—A drug from the plant *Cannabis sativa;* leaves and flower tops are smoked or eaten.

media—All the various means of communication used to inform, entertain or influence people; includes advertising, newspapers, radio, magazines, movies, music, music videos, TV shows, websites, computer games, blogs, podcasts and social media.

medicine—A drug given for prevention, diagnosis or treatment of disease.

merchandise—Goods or other things that are bought and sold.

minors—People who are under full legal age.

misuse—To use improperly.

motivation—A willingness or strong intent to do something.

nausea—A sick feeling in the stomach, with an impulse to vomit.

negative—Harmful or destructive.

negative influence—Something that has an effect that is not positive or constructive, or one that is harmful.

nicotine—A powerful chemical and toxic poison found in the tobacco plant, especially in the leaves; the chief addictive drug in tobacco.

norms—The beliefs and behaviors shared by and accepted within a group.

outcome—Result or consequence.

over-the-counter drug—A legal drug used for self-medication that can be bought without a prescription.

peers—People of the same age or close in age who are similar in many ways.

perceived norms—What people think others are doing or believe.

percentage—A given number out of every hundred.

Health Terms Glossary

(continued)

pharmacist—A medical professional licensed to prepare and dispense prescription drugs.

physical—Having to do with the body and its functions.

pledge—A promise a person makes to themselves and/or others.

policy—An official statement or position on an issue that often sets forth rules or guidelines for individual or group actions and outlines consequences for breaking these rules.

positive influence—Something that has a beneficial or helpful effect.

possession—Something one has or owns; specifically, having a drug on one's person or in one's home or vehicle.

prescription—A written request from a doctor that a drug be given to a patient by a pharmacist.

pressure—Any influence that pushes or urges someone to do something.

rebel—To resist authority.

recruit—To get people to join a group or organization or take a specific action.

reinforce—To strengthen by adding something new.

reproductive system—The organs involved in sexual activity and creating offspring.

resist—To fight against, oppose or refuse to go along with.

responsibility—Something a person is required or has committed to do.

risk—The likelihood of injury, damage or other negative results following an action or behavior.

roleplay—An activity in which people are given an example situation and practice their responses to learn a skill such as refusals or conflict resolution.

scavenger hunt—A game in which players or teams have to find and gather certain objects or information.

secondhand smoke—The smoke given off by the burning end of a cigarette, pipe or cigar, and the smoke exhaled from the lungs of smokers.

self-image—The view a person has of themselves.

self-talk—The ideas a person thinks or says to themselves.

short term—Happening right away.

smokeless tobacco—Tobacco products that are placed in the mouth or sniffed into the nose rather than burned or smoked.

social—Having to do with living or being with others.

Health Terms Glossary

(continued)

sponsorship—When people or companies provide money to help put on an event. In exchange their names or products are featured in ads at these events.

stages—Periods or levels in a process of development.

stimulant—A drug that speeds up the central nervous system.

target—The object of an attack or criticism; the person information or advertising is intended to reach.

testimonial—A statement recommending a person or product.

tobacco—The leaves of plants from the genus *Nicotiana* and the products made from these leaves, such as cigarettes, cigars, smokeless tobacco and vaping juices.

tolerance—When the body adapts to a drug; results in the need for an increased dose to feel the same effects.

vape device—A device that heats up a liquid to create an aerosol that users breathe in.

vaping—Using a vape device to inhale an aerosol containing flavors, nicotine and other chemicals.

withdrawal—Symptoms that occur when users who are dependent on a drug stop taking it.